VOLUNTARY EUTHANASIA—
IS THERE AN ALTERNATIVE?

Voluntary Euthanasia–
Is there an Alternative?

by Duncan W. Vere

C.M.F. Publications

First Published — 1971
Second Edition, revised and enlarged — 1979

Duncan W. Vere, M.D., F.R.C.P., is Professor of Therapeutics in the University of London and Consultant Physician. To this second edition has been added Appendix I on the present legal position in relation to Euthanasia, contributed by Nick Miller, M.A., M.Sc.

Price £1.00

SBN 85111 938 7

Printed by Stanley L. Hunt (Printers) Ltd. Rushden Northamptonshire

Contents

6. Euthanasia is concerned with laws—
   - Present British law
   - The effect of weakening law
   - Need the law prohibit mercy-killing?

7. The liberal principle—
   - The case against prohibition
   - The case against acceptance—
     - (a) Adequate safeguards cannot be achieved
     - (b) Conservative attitudes to life would be weakened
     - (c) Humane pre-terminal care is a preferable and practical alternative
   - Further theistic objections—
     - (a) Theism commends itself to reason
     - (b) Liberty is curbed by evil
     - (c) Life-taking without a mandate is wrong

8. Who would perform Euthanasia?—
   - Inevitable medical involvement
   - A damaged professional relationship
   - A divided profession

9. What would be the alternative?

10. Conclusion

Appendix 1 Recent Proposals for Changes in the English Criminal Law Relating to Euthanasia and Kindred Offences
By Nick Miller, M.A., M.Sc.

Appendix II An Argument from the Theory of Knowledge

Appendix III An Argument from Modern Theology

References

Introduction

Interest grows in the control of death. Man, noting that much fear and suffering stems from ignorance, has set out in quest of new knowledge. In this quest, many causes of human pain have been recognised, isolated, understood and mastered. Not content with learning to control external problems—weather, flood, beasts or microbes—man has tackled the problems within—ignorance, superstition, disease and crime. Inevitably the journey has led him on to seek to control his own life, its beginnings and its pains. Now a short step forward brings him face to face with the last enemy, ageing and death.

But all along this hazardous road of developing health care there have been no clear cut ethical stopping places where it was easy to say, 'thus far and no further'. So why should we expect such clear cut issues now? If every ethical decision then seemed at first to be indistinct, and progress was hard fought, why should we expect to find anything different now? Inevitably birth and death are now under scrutiny. Birth-control is advocated as an answer to the starvation and over-crowding facing the human race. Should death-control also be attempted?

The practical method for death-control, which is increasingly considered, is 'Voluntary Euthanasia'. Euthanasia (literally death without suffering) means any way to make death easy, but the word has now been restricted to mean death induced in order to terminate suffering in incurable diseases. This aim, and the belief that recovery is impossible, should be shared by the sufferer and euthanasiast alike. The present suggestion is neither for compulsory, nor even generally practised Euthanasia, but for a legal permission to be given to those who accept the method to practise it. In all that follows, 'Euthanasia' will be understood to mean the method and intent just defined, unless the word be otherwise qualified. However, it should be noted that neither the 'voluntary' aspect, nor the near prospect of a natural but painful death, is a necessary entailment of the concept. Some, but not all, proponents of Euthanasia would support compulsory Euthanasia, or Euthanasia for non-fatal but disabling disorders.

The proponents of Euthanasia marshal three main arguments in their favour—*freedom* of the individual to choose death, the assumed 'right to die', *compassion*, and *progress*.

Since the problem is very complex, it is difficult to gain much from a discussion which treats it as a whole from the start. It seems better to discuss parts of the problem as they develop from each other in a logical order. This we have tried to do. Compassion is discussed in section 4, freedom in section 7, and progress in section 9.

Before ethical problems are discussed some basic misconceptions must be cleared away. In this booklet we have tried to give a closely reasoned debate on some of the primary ethical, legal and practical arguments about euthanasia. For more practical and clinical discussions the reader should refer to Twycross (1978) and Saunders (1978). A central theme is now 'the right to die', by which some used to mean the right to have one's life ended in certain circumstances, but which has now been broadened to include much more the assumed right to be *allowed* to die from natural causes. This broader view is particularly discussed by Ruth Russell (1977). Because the law is now so important in relation to this whole subject, a new Appendix I has been added in this 1979 edition of the present book by Nick Miller. He shows how attempts are being made to legitimise various forms of assisted suicide or to prevent unnecessary treatment.

1. Euthanasia and the concept of death

When is death? The simple definition of death, acceptable for many generations, is now difficult to accept because new knowledge has forced us to redefine life. Ordinary descriptions of life reflect the fact that it is organised at many different levels of complexity. There is molecular, subcellular, cellular, organ, system, corporeal, mental and, for those who accept the idea, spiritual life, and therefore death can also be defined in each of these sets of terms. Most of the cells which line the gut live for only one or two days. Because they are continually renewed, the tract remains alive. It then contributes to the total life of the person whose gut it is. If much of the tract died say because he took a corrosive poison, he might linger on 'alive' for a few days, but towards the end of that time (when hypotension and metabolic changes ensued) he might become permanently unresponsive, mentally dead, despite persistence of heart beat and breathing. These would not necessarily mean that he was 'alive', only that two systems, cardiovascular and respiratory, still functioned. They could continue to do so, in other circumstances, for many months after his cerebrum was dead and beyond recovery.

Legal definitions have to be unequivocal because they are needed to lead to unambiguous decisions. Pulse and breathing seem handy, unequivocal signs of life. In times when death happened quickly, and nearly all at once, they were all that was needed. Now that death has become, through medical science, a graded process, they are about as relevant to its definition as would be a flashing light at the rear of a crashed car a sign that it could be driven away!

A new definition of death is required; it can be obtained

only by redefining life. We would suggest that "human life is the ability, actual *or in potential*, to respond to others or to be self-aware". Human death is then "all other states of organisation or disorganisation". This definition is based on cerebral function. It conforms to the idea that life is a subjective thing, so that a wide margin must always be left for error in actual decisions. This is because observers cannot always estimate potential, or record evidence of self-awareness or response.

The definition leads at once to the problem and possibility of varieties of 'mental death'. For example it is conceivable that the evidences for mental death might be temporary, or that psychiatric changes could be so severe as to become tantamount to death despite organic integrity of brain function. Since mental death, too, may be difficult to determine (even by highly trained specialists using complex equipment) ample room must be left for *potential*, and respect accorded to any doubtful 'lives'. It seems best to reserve the idea of death for situations where there is no cerebral response or future possibility of it. This excludes all cases where responses are present, but are disordered, however severely.

The chief objective criterion available to demonstrate cerebral function is, in the unconscious subject, the electro-encephalogram. Silverman and others (1969) showed the remarkable reliability of this test in 1,600 cases; provided only that care and competence be used in making the test and in ensuring that drug effects, metabolic diseases and hypothermia are excluded. Recently, these tests have been further elaborated, and a set of precise methods have been agreed upon and are the official policy of the Department of Health (Brit. Med.J. 1978).

If opposition to Euthanasia is based on outmoded definitions of life, these definitions are uninformed and should be dismissed. So should efforts to convince people that we already practise Euthanasia in those cases where, after cerebral death has been confirmed, the other functions are allowed to 'die' as therapy is withdrawn. To withdraw therapy after the brain has died is not Euthanasia; it is not the deliberate, requested, extinction of the living. Cerebral and personal deaths coincide, and have, if our definition is followed, already occurred when therapy is withdrawn. Nor, to look at it the other way round, is it right to struggle for bodily existence after the brain has died on the grounds that to fail to do this would amount to Euthanasia. Sadly, both of the serious confusions just described are common. They have all been perpetrated recently by informed and experienced people (cf. Joseph Fletcher, 1969, and Lord Platt, 1970, p. 660) and as long as they persist there can be no clear appraisal of the problem.

2. Euthanasia implies a death which ends incurable suffering

Sudden deaths, and illnesses which cause little suffering, are not the concern of the proponents of Euthanasia; nor is suffering in the course of remediable illness. Those who support Euthanasia are concerned with incurable, distressing maladies before the stage of impending death. What is never specified, because it cannot be, is the severity of disability which could be deemed to justify Euthanasia. Usually it is taken as extreme disability, but it is noteworthy that an 'irremediable condition' as defined in the Voluntary Euthanasia Bill of 1969 could have comprised almost any chronic, serious ailment, or indeed normal ageing itself! It has been hinted from the start of the Voluntary Euthanasia Legalisation society, that to suffer a sense of uselessness could, in time, constitute adequate grounds for Euthanasia (e.g. Listowel, 1969, pp. 6-7, Wolbarst, 1939 quoting Charlotte Gilman).

At present, most are likely to concur that a 'therapeutic' course so extreme as to court or accelerate death could be considered only in demonstrably hopeless illness (Yale Kamisar, 1969, p. 87). The problem then is how to prove an illness to be hopeless. Both opponents (Yale Kamisar, 1969, p. 87) and proponents (Gresham, 1969, p. 151; Williams, 1957, p. 283) of Euthanasia legislation agree that medical prognostic error is inevitable, even given accurate diagnosis, which itself is beyond our powers to guarantee. One writer seemed to surprise even himself with the discovery that a full half of all doctors are below average competence! (See the discussion by Yale Kamisar, 1969, pp. 98-105.) All human efforts, however carefully made, are subject to measurable error (Vere, 1963) and it is safe to assume that errors in prognosis would occur.

Two points then arise, of ascending importance:

(i) *Prognostic error.* The proponents of Euthanasia seek to evade the problem of prognostic error by asserting that errors are either few (Millard, 1931, pp. 701, 717), comparatively unimportant (Flew, 1969, p. 40; Gresham, 1969, p. 151) or inevitable in all proper forms of human activity (Williams, 1957, p. 283). Each argument is a special plea, for errors in Euthanasia would be doubly different from other errors. Firstly they would be irretrievable with respect to life, and secondly they would be incorrigible in the sense that the sufferer could never furnish evidence about the success or appropriateness of his 'treatment'. This being so, their low number (impossible to ascertain or establish), their unimportance compared to other errors (common grounds for comparison do not exist), and their inevitablity cannot be said to mitigate their gravity but, if anything, make it worse. Error in Euthanasia would be qualitatively very much greater than errors in other medical fields; the tragedy to just one person killed in error should discourage anyone from Euthanasia. Everyone has an irremediable disease as soon as he is born, which shows obvious physical signs at some time between the ages of 40 and 60. The real thrust of prognostic uncertainty is not merely that some may die by mistake. It is that everyone, at least if over 40, is in principle a candidate for Euthanasia if these ideas are followed to their logical end.

It is curious that some argue from the same premises (of the few cases for whom a law is needed, and the gravity of diagnostic errors) *for* Euthanasia, but *against* capital punishment! Granted, one is 'voluntary', the other society's compulsion; but we should not argue that a tragedy enforced by society is greater than one which results from someone's mistaken request. This argument does not close the case against Euthanasia, any more than it does against capital punishment, but it does urge an extremely conservative and careful approach which is not in evidence amongst all proponents of Euthanasia.

(ii) The second point about prognostic error is the most important of all. Euthanasia, of necessity, *presupposes hopelessness.* The proponent of Euthanasia must suppose that there is a fully useless state of life (Alexander, 1949, p. 116) a distress which human kindness and medical skill cannot reduce a disease which is certain to kill (Barrington, 1969). This view runs counter to the remarkable hopefulness of the Christian message, and cannot be squared with fact. However, this must be balanced by the obvious facts that the Christian faith does not expect life on earth to go on for ever, and accepts death as a natural part of life. So, it is not a Christian objective to fight off death at all costs. It is the rejection of hopelessness, conserving what may be left of life, whilst accepting death, that is characteristically Christian.

Everyone feels useless at times, but there is no sentient, or potentially sentient person who has nothing to contribute, no disease which has never remitted, no condition which cannot be substantially relieved by human aid, and no prognosis which is never wrongly made. The Christian view is, by contrast, one of hope and of care, one which links the weakening of this life with progress towards the next. Euthanasia springs from hopelessness and despair. It is not, therefore, a natural companion of Christianity, but is radically opposed to it in the direction of its motive and practice.

3. Euthanasia is death acceleration

The speeding of death is a source of serious confusion in many writings on Euthanasia. A leading feature of the debate has been failure to discriminate between the ways in which death may be brought forward, a failure which has been freely exploited by spokesmen for or against the practice.

Distinct situations

It is not difficult, in fact, to distinguish about a dozen distinct therapeutic situations which differ in their ethical content. The main classification, however, separates cases where (1) therapy was omitted by reason of uncertainty of its effects, (2) cases where therapy was given to relieve distress and happened to accelerate death, and (3) cases where medical intervention was designed to bring death forward. Many examples of direct confusion of these categories may be found in the writings of proponents of Euthanasia (e.g. Gillon, 1969, pp. 173, 191; G. P. Fletcher, 1969, p. 76), a confusion which is easier to sustain when life is defined on a corporeal basis, rather than by cerebral function.

It seems that many people find it difficult to accept two things: (i) that *all* medical and surgical therapies may at times *shorten* life rather than prolong it, and (ii) that no doctor or nurse can be expected to persist with a treatment which they do not believe to be helping their patient. For example, one has only to consider amputation for gangrene in an elderly person to see that life may be shortened as easily as it may be prolonged by surgery, and that a surgeon may reverse his decision to operate should the patient, for example, get a chest infection.

Each of the first two categories above may be sub-divided into cases where the risk to life could not be foreseen in detail, and those where it was well known, but reckoned to be justified. The discussions, particularly by lawyers, about the problem of withholding treatment, particularly when made by non-medical people, seem almost always to lack recognition of the fact that *all* treatments involve a balanced assessment of profits and risks, and of omissions as well as commissions (see e.g. G. P. Fletcher, 1969, p. 75). It is presumably because people do not understand the nature of medical treatment that the law singles out cases of terminal care from all the others when it is argued that to withhold active treatment (aimed at cure) is Euthanasia.

If omission of therapy, because it may diminish a patient's brain function, is a guilty act, then by the same token may *any* medical treatment be held to be negligent in that sense (see particularly Giertz 1966). The unrealistic complexities of legal interpretation here are well shown by G. P. Fletcher's discussion of an omitted insulin injection (1969, p. 82). (It seems, according to Fletcher, that the law would make a difference between insulin shots and mechanical ventilation on the grounds of 'contemporary standards' regarding their use. Fortunately, biology is not subject to these standards. The problems which surround omission of either form of treatment are biologically one and the same, whether the law or the public thinks so or not.)

If it is to be insisted that a doctor *must* persist with what he takes to be an ineffective remedy because it *might* be effective, or because it is conventional therapy for that illness in terms of contemporary standards, or whatever, then his therapy is reduced to a mindless automatism.

Each of these separable types of case which we are discussing can be further sub-divided into those cases where the patient consented to an act, and those where he did not; those where he was ignorant of s portent and those where he had given prior, if not immediate, consent.

Deliberate death acceleration

One category stands out as distinct—when death is willed—the distinction being one of motive. This is 'Euthanasia' in the modern sense; it comprises the 'voluntary' variety when requested by the sufferer, 'involuntary Euthanasia' if it is against his wish. There is also the most dubiously definable category 'voluntary by prior consent', if a patient has left some written request to that effect. These are all distinguishable situations with different shades of ethical difficulty.

Two further special cases now merit comment. There is the familiar 'switching off' problem, the withholding of therapy in case of proven brain death which we have shown to be freely confused with Euthanasia. We have already argued that these should be distinguished sharply on the grounds of the definition of life. This case is surely an example of the first category discussed above, viz. omission of a therapy which is unlikely to help, despite a known risk to corporeal life. This seems a preferable distinction to that which designates this process as 'indirect Euthanasia' (Fletcher, J., 1969, pp. 66-68) a term which suggests an affinity with 'direct Euthanasia' far too close to match the reality. 'Indirect Euthanasia' is a verbal innuendo which is highly misleading.

Another distinct problem is when a choice arises between a highly risky treatment (which may prove fatal in a substantial proportion of cases, but which may also conserve mental function should it succeed) and a less life-risking therapy, which has less chance of preserving the mind. Such choices may confront a neurosurgeon, for example, when dealing with brain tumours.

It is important to note how wide a play of possible mechanisms and motives exists within nature's repertoire of ways to bring life to a close, whether life support is temporarily gained from a machine or not, there is amply room for a wide variety of natural mechanisms, and of medical motives too. But the confused discussions of the subject often end as if there can be only one desirable, kind and effective therapy for the incurably sick—voluntary Euthanasia—and the suggestion that this is cruelly denied by existing laws. We would argue that the omission of the therapy which is effective only for the body, and not for the dying mind is, and always has been, a part of good medical practice. Ethical and practical objections do, however, abound where therapy is omitted (or used) *negligently*, or where there is *intent to end life*, whether sentient or potentially sentient, whatever the 'quality' of that sentience may be.

A final question to explore in this section is how, in each of the distinct circumstances just described, *death might be accelerated 'voluntarily'*. First let it be said that no ethical problem is seen in a previously expressed wish not to be resuscitated should irreparable brain damage occur. But the proponents of 'voluntary Euthanasia' presuppose a candidate of 'responsible' mind (Explanatory Memorandum, 1969, clause 4) who is under some intolerable suffering which is reasonably "expected to cause him severe distress or render him incapable of rational existence". (Section 1.2 of the Voluntary Euthanasia Bill 1969.) Since both subjective qualifications (responsible mind and severe distress or irrational existence) can scarcely be held to coexist, it must be presumed that either the candidate volunteers in view of *future* distress, or he volunteers in a mind disturbed by present distress. How can a man decide the degree of distress that he is likely to tolerate at some future date? Who is to measure it when it occurs? When he is distressed, and then signs a form, can his judgment be regarded as natural? In effect, this comes back to the need to rely on the *doctor's* judgment in each case, made at the time of the actual illness, but in the light of all that he knows about the patient. It is hard to see how a balanced 'voluntary' judgment can ever be attained, whether the suffering is now distorting the patient's mind, or is a prospect of future horror to him.

Four *practical examples* may aid this discussion. The writer knows accurately of a man who endured so much during two resuscitations that he asked (should cardiac arrest recur) that he be allowed to die. The arrest recurred, but he was again revived by a passer-by who was unaware of his request. Two years later the patient was at the centre of a happy family, apparently in perfect health, and had forgotten the distress of his resuscitation.

Again, at a debate in Cambridge the issue was won by neither speaker, but by the chairman, a distinguished professor, who said that he had been so badly burned in youth that a hopeless prognosis had been given. So intense had been his pain that he would have gladly accepted Euthanasia had it been available to him.

The writer also cared for a woman in respiratory failure who, after several days' intensive care withdrew her endotracheal tube with the balloon inflated in order to remark that she had "had enough of tubes", and "why did we not just write her off?" Intensive care was stopped forthwith. It so happened that she survived. Later, she recollected none of the therapy, but thanked everyone cordially for it, because she said "I suppose it must have saved my life".

The only patient who has ever asked the writer to be 'put to death' by a dose was clearly confused. He was given a phenothiazine derivative, and, after a few hours of thinking he was dead, forgot the whole episode. Next day he had become more orientated and was sitting up by the window happily remarking about the sunshine!

These are not just hard, exceptional cases which make bad laws. It is in the nature of the problem that judgment is impaired by intense suffering—or the imagined prospect of it. Prior requests may be made under duress of circumstances, if not of pain. The 'I' who wishes Euthanasia now, in calm consciousness, might prefer another course later were that calm preserved on into an illness. But so often it is lost, withdrawing from the sufferer any hope of retraction and rendering the unconfirmed avowals of yesterday of doubtful value.

In short there is no such thing as a true 'voluntary Euthanasia'. Paradoxically, if mercy is to be the motive, most of those who 'need' Euthanasia are incapable of 'voluntary' assent, the dements and the insane. Equally vulnerable will be those who ask for it because they are depressed, confused, paranoid or frightened; or are aware of pressure from relatives, real or imagined; or just feel that they are in the way.

Doctors' decisions

Put in another way, doctors have long worked in the confidence that recovery is what their patient would have wanted had he been of sound mind and able to choose at the time he became ill. It has, then, always seemed right to strive for recovery whenever it seemed attainable, even when a patient's wishes could not be heard. But it cannot seem right, when dealing with such people, to think that they might (if at that time of sound mind) have chosen *not* to recover, and then to act on this untestable idea. There are even times when, as in the case of burning just described, doctors would normally decide to override a patient's wish to die, and work for his recovery. To summarise, a moment of dispassionate choice can never coincide with the intolerable suffering to which it is directed. This, compounded with frequent prognostic uncertainties, imposes insoluble problems for the euthanasiast.

4. The ethical difficulties of death acceleration

It is essential to think about the rightness and practicability of Euthanasia. Were it both wrong and inexpedient, or just agreed to be wrong, no case for its practice would exist. Even so, we should not let the matter rest there. We should aim to find other acceptable methods to relieve the sufferings of those who die in severe pain. Were it right, but inexpedient, it would be necessary only to discover better methods. If it were clearly right and expedient it would long since have become the common practice of mankind.

The propriety of assisting suicide. The Euthanasia problem centres about assisting suicide. The concept is often presented by opponents as if Euthanasia were murder, on the straightforward assumption that the 6th commandment applies equally to all killings, which are equally culpable. But 'murder', by definition, requires a guilty intent (in law, a *mens rea*), whereas Euthanasia is designed to be merciful.

The real issue is whether we shall practise life control by means of suicide. Strong attempts are being made to mould public attitudes so as to be more favourable to suicide (Barrington, 1969, p. 156; Listowel, 1969, p. 7). It is no exaggeration to say that some wish to popularise suicide as a respectable end to insoluble problems, whether medical or social.

Public attitudes to suicide

Three arguments are in vogue, all specious in various ways. It is first argued that public disapproval of suicide stems from faulty traditions attributable to Christianity, an attitude of harsh condemnation of suicide which ill befits those who believe in '*mors janua vitae*' (death is the gateway to life). True, there have been over-harsh condemnations, as there have been of drunkenness. But that in itself makes no fault commendable. It is an old trick to whitewash an evil by revealing errors in those who oppose it.

The next argument is that the 1961 Suicide Act, by lifting penalties, disclosed a new attitude to public toleration, or even approval of suicide, as a means of problem solving (on this 'new attitude' see Listowel, 1969, p. 5; Matthews, 1969, p. 27; Barrington, 1969, p. 153; Clark-Kennedy, 1969, p. 152). But the Act was framed to provide mercy, not social approval, towards a would-be suicide. Suicide is now not a crime. Of course even if suicide were legal, which it still is not, a legal act can be immoral. (Lord Longford, 1969, columns 1189, 1193.)

Lastly, and most confusingly, the examples of Oates, Damien or even Jesus Christ are advanced as acts of voluntary life surrender for the sake of others. (Flew, 1969, pp. 43-47; Kamisar, 1969, pp. 86-87; Soper, 1969, column 1198; Clark-Kennedy, 1969, p. 152). At first this argument seems attractive for it makes suicide ennobling. Unhappily closer study shows it to be largely irrelevant. None of these three men committed suicide; each took a deliberate step in accepting death as an act of faith in God to meet the need of their fellow men. None invited help to shorten their life; each surrendered life to forces outside himself. Each died not for their own sake, but because they were engaged in work on the behalf of others. None of them seems to have wished to end his own pain, or an incurable disease, or to escape from anything. None of these factors applies to ordinary requests for Euthanasia. It does not help to try to link Euthanasia with examples of heroic self sacrifice. These examples bear no true resemblance to Euthanasia.

Of course, nothing we have said proves that suicide should not be approved on other grounds, but only that the current arguments designed to secure its approval are irrelevant. The 1961 Act in fact retained penalties for assisting suicide, so that it is indeed difficult to argue that this Act reflects social approval of the practice.

Religious contributions to the ethical debate

It is frequently urged that religious argument should be deleted from serious discussion of Euthanasia (see e.g. Gresham, 1969, p. 151). The book to which Gresham contributed opened with Yeat's poem:

> Nor dread nor hope attend
> A dying animal
> A man awaits his end
> Dreading and hoping all.

Presumably this quotation must have been set there either to argue that man should be treated like the animals, or conversely, to show the relevance of religious argument, since it is this which determines the difference between man and beast. (See by all means the debate between Lords Allwyn and Chudleigh, 1969, cols. 1186, 1209.) Religion *is* a part of man. It does colour all his attitudes. It cannot but be discussed.

The Christian and Atheist standpoints are more opposed on this issue than any others in Britain today. (Most theistic beliefs coincide to some extent on the problem of suicide, but only Christian theism will be discussed, since the writer is not competent to consider the views of other faiths.) Both views desire the best for sufferers, both admit that there are areas of uncertainty over what is best. The Atheist, regarding man as master of his fate, and God as non-existent or unknowable, stresses what man has already learnt in order to prove human self-sufficiency. The Christian, by contrast, stresses man's objective weakness, need and limitations, and their remedy as God's revealed word and work. He is therefore usually more aware than others of human limitations in decisions about life.

We need not discuss Humanist objections to suicide, for they are determined wholly locally, by the situation where they arise. There is no absolute objection to suicide (Flew, 1969, pp. 43-45; Barrington, 1969, p. 153), which is at times strongly approved. However, purely pragmatic utilitarian arguments of seemingly equal strength can be made for and against Euthanasia (see the debate between Kamisar and Williams, 1969). This, if anything, adds to the theistic view that man's unaided strength cannot lead him to solve such issues.

Three Christian objections

There seem to be three main Christian objections to suicide. These will be explained in detail and a positive statement of the Christian alternative used to end this section.

(a) *The 'image of God'*. In Genesis chapter 9, and in many other places, it is clearly explained that man differs from animals in his creation 'in God's image'. It is added that, for this reason, his life merits extreme respect. Innocent life should, in general, never be taken. This does not merely mean that life-taking with guilty intent is forbidden; it also implies that an account of the disposal of all lives will be required of man by God. This idea is the source of the 'sanctity of life' attitude, which easily degenerates in human currency into a rule which is thoughtlessly applied. It is nowhere stated that the preservation of human life transends *all* other considerations, only that it is among the most important considerations. However, it is necessary to say that because the 'image of God' doctrine is broader than the case of murder, and comprises man's answerability for human life, it has been heavily attacked by those who favour Euthanasia or abortion (Cf. 'The Sanctity of Life and the Criminal Law,' by Williams). If it were right for a man to take his own life, it would probably be right for someone else to assist him, or for him to ask for this. So the 'image of God' idea applies directly to suicide attempted by someone of sane mind.

Many theologians feel that the 'image of God' doctrine presents an absolute bar to suicide in and of itself. Whether or not one takes that view, it must be conceded that it does stand right across the Atheist's view that the value of a man's life is determinable solely by himself or his fellows. It certainly proves that some Divine mandate is needed to take human life in any way. It could be argued that, if 'man in God's image' means anything, it is that he is endowed with rational choice, which could include that of ending his own life. But this is never the context of the doctrine in Scripture, even by those who most needed that sort of 'help' and who best knew the meaning of the doctrine, for example, Job, David, Jeremiah or Christ. It is surely most significant that its context in Genesis 9 *is* a prohibition against killing man. It was, in fact, only the view of an apostate, King Saul, that suicide was a helpful option. The example of Christ, who is particularly described as the outstanding 'man in God's image', is most noteworthy. He knew death. He submitted to it knowingly. He believed it could be right to die for others (Matthew 10.24-39). He cannot have been unaware of Greek suicide customs (Gillon, 1969, p. 176). He was only too deeply aware of the extreme of human misery, particularly of those contemporaries whom, like modern Atheists, He could not heal because they would not trust Him. He was not a man who feared to canvas new or unpopular views if they were right. He knew that murder implied malice (Matthew 5), and that there were killings devoid of malice. He was always eager to show that the mere prolongation of existence was not man's highest good (Matthew 24.9). He had the means to commit or advocate suicide, had many friends who might in the modern view have 'benefited' from it (and the ancient world would have been agog had He done it). But there is nothing to show that He even considered suicide as an option, even when it might have seemed most desirable (cf. Matthew 10.27).

In this light, Gillon's contention (1969, p. 176f.) that opposition to suicide is a relatively late Christian importation, and that the practice was never condemned by Christ, is particularly naive. (All formalised doctrine is a relatively recent importation, simply because doctrines tended to be codified some centuries after their origins.) The cardinal fact is that since Euthanasia was known, had Christ or His apostles failed to support it as a widely practised, merciful pagan custom to which they had no objection, they might have seemed guilty of marked hypocrisy. They did not advocate suicide because they were too busy ministering a satisfying alternative, and presumably because they did object to it. Christ, the true image of God, did not take His life into His own hands, but committed it to God to whom it belonged. It was left to Judas to explore the alternatives. Christian concern is always *for* life and living relationships.

(b) '*Divine Providence*'

> Frail children of dust, and feeble as frail,
> In Thee do we trust, nor find Thee to fail,
> Thy mercies how tender, how firm to the end,
> Our Maker, Defender, Redeemer and Friend.

It is no surprise that the attitudes of some modern Christians on suicide are ambiguous, for the doctrine of 'providence' is one of the most neglected in their contemporary religious expliqué of life. There is not space here to restate it, though reference must be made to Calvin's penetrating account (Institutes, Book 1, chs. 15, 16 and 17). He shows, from a very broad review of Scriptures, that life is God's gift, and its end to be determined by Him, at least so far as His own servants are concerned. This in no way prevents the use of curative means, which are themselves shown to be part of the providential gift.

Though the argument of 'an allotted span' appears in

Scripture the emphasis is not that God's most tenacious ambition is to ensure that we all live for a certain number of days! This, stated in that crude form, would clearly interdict curative medicine (see Matthews, 1969, p. 26). The emphasis instead seems to be that God, whilst giving to us a mandate to heal by natural means, withholds from us the right to decide how long someone should live.

Of suicide, Calvin wrote, "those who have learned this modesty (i.e. the modest acknowledgment of God's providential overruling in their lives) will neither murmur against God for adversity in time past, nor charge Him with the blame of their own wickedness . . . on the other hand, they will not like the Youth in Plautus, destroy themselves in despair, as if hurried away by the Fates. . . . They will rather enquire and learn from Scripture what is pleasing to God, and then, under the guidance of the Spirit, endeavour to attain it." "If the Lord has marked the moment of our death, it cannot be escaped, it is vain to toil and use precaution . . . these are all vain remedies, laid hold of to correct the will of God, or His certain decree does not fix the limits of life and death . . . and other matters which men, according as they desire and hate, study by their own industry to secure or avoid."

This quotation is made to show the temper of Calvin's distillation from Scripture. There is no space for detailed argument here, though the serious student should refer to the wide range of verses to which he alluded. In short, his interpretation was that all decisions should be made with reference to God's revealed will. Some, it has been revealed, are not open for man to take, including the decisions to end his own life. It seems that a Christian who believes in providence will be unlikely to support suicide, whilst one who does not will remain in doubt. Atheists, no doubt, will be untroubled by any of this debate.

It is important, while discussing providence, to think of life as God's gift. As Calvin quickly showed, this includes all of life, suffering as well as joy, pains as well as comforts. Whether they accept 'providence' or not, all Christians agree that suffering can become as much God's opportunity as health, though it is not to be courted or prolonged so that the opportunity can be extended. (Those who have espoused this last argument, when of sound mind, seem to have wanted the ennobling benefits of suffering for other people rather than for themselves!)

It is obvious that suffering so extreme as to distort the mind and destroy personality is excluded here. The Christian obligation there, as in lesser pains, is to bring effective relief. That said, it is a fact, though, that many incurable illnesses have been for countless people, Christian or not, opportunities for a full reorientation of their view of life rather than for suicide. The Christian, further to this, often finds suffering an opportunity for witness and amendment of life. If redemption cannot, here and now, begin to reshape *all* aspects of real life, it is worth less than Christians customarily assert. Christ showed how suffering can be used. We cannot follow Him in that use, but can emulate His attitudes. Certainly, it is an anti-Christian argument that suffering is always to be evaded by choice, still less by suicide. Suffering is not to be sought either, nor can it always furnish redemptive opportunities. We are merely stating the objective truth that, since *some* sufferings can be turned to good use, no-one should say that *all* suffering should be escaped. The element of suicide which is in radical opposition to Christianity is its despair.

This leads on to the statement that there is in the certainty of God's providence the uncertainty of physical prognosis. (This is not being stated here as an observable fact, which would seem to be true, but rather as a constituent part of providence.) Calvin showed, in a very helpful section (Institutes, Chapter XVII, pages 195-196) that God's 'repentance' is not an arbitrary change of mind but a deliberate, pre-planned, change of action following some foreseen choice on a sufferer's part. For this reason, Christians are reluctant to speak of 'terminal illness'. Relief may come when other circumstances change in a sufferer's life. Hezekiah is a good Old Testament example of someone who believed himself to be dying but found after prayer that he was to live for some years.

These words are written with feeling. For at the very moment of writing a woman who was admitted to hospital moribund, and declared by a distinguished expert in her complaint to be so beyond aid as to need no more investigation, has recovered. She had seemed to have irreversible renal failure for two or three weeks. When the nature of her problem was explained to her and to her family, they prayed and a year's recovery followed. We do not claim this as a miracle; it is only the sort of thing a Christian might expect to happen at times to those whose work is not yet done. It is what might be expected from the doctrine of Providence. The argument applies equally to the ungodly, whose demand for suicide affirms his atheism, so making it forever impossible for him to obtain evidence of the Providence he declines to recognise.

(*c*) *Shared motives in assisted suicide*

In the use of restorative therapy it can be safely assumed to be right to treat someone positively whatever his motives may happen to be. For example, were medicine requested by a criminal who was determined to exploit his renewed health in a life of crime, it is clearly the doctor's duty to treat him, and to leave to the patient the decision of what to do with his health. So the positive good of therapy prevails in independence of the recipient's motives.

Now, with Euthanasia this is no longer the case, and a practical objection arises. A Christian, even one who may be liberally disposed to Euthanasia, may be asked to assist suicide. He cannot ascertain whether the candidate's motive is plausible, and so has no means to decide the validity of his decision to end life, or not, as the case may be. He has no means of telling whether or not he *should* agree to the patient's motive in asking for the means of suicide. Why should there be this difference? It is simply a question of *authority*. Christians believe in general that they have a mandate to heal, but no authority to dispose of life. (The point is perhaps more easily seen if one considers what whould happen if a doctor let the criminal die because he was a criminal. He would have no authority to do that.) This problem does not arise in healing, restorative therapy. The doctor's duty is clear. It is to heal, and to leave the decision of what to do with health to the patient.

Analogous problems have always existed in medicine, whenever its role has not been therapeutic in the traditional sense of that term. Plastic surgery may be used to evade justice, sterilisation to cheat a marital partner, and drugs to modify social behaviour. In each the problem of motive sharing arises between doctor and patient.

If Euthanasia is to share with traditional healing this remarkable immunity from motivational critique, it must be proved to be a 'therapy' in the traditional sense. If this is not so, it will suffer from ethical counter pressures. It cannot, in fact, ever be a therapy in that way; though it aims to relieve suffering, it removes all hope of conserving health and, as has been shown, signifies that the doctor accedes not to some universally agreed mandate to heal, but to a patient's individual wish to end his life. It is possible to relieve suffering in other ways, methods which do not irrevocably damage life. They are true 'therapies'. Euthanasia is not.

Many will say that motives cannot be assessed, that a Christian is called upon not to judge others' motives. This is to argue that responsibility for a therapy is solely the patient's, not the practitioner's. This attitude has led to an astonishing cynicism about professional ethics. Mr. Justice Ormrod argued that doctors have only two alternatives. They can bow to social pressures for life-manipulating operations, or abdicate in favour of a state-run cadre of technicians (Ormrod, 1968). It was similarly argued that a gynaecologist asked by other doctors to perform abortion *should* not add his own opinion (Williams, 1970). But a professional, who unquestioningly shares social motivation, has in so doing become less than a technician. He is less than a morally responsible man.

Certainly, he is no longer a professional, whose function is to give informed advice in what he judges to be the interests of his client. It has even been argued that, since the Geneva Code forbids a doctor to allow religion to affect his judgment on treatment, he must not allow his religious views to influence his decisions on abortions. In this cynical way a Code which was intended to protect patients and doctors from each others' prejudices which could damage health, is being twisted disingenuously till it comes to mean that the customer is always right. The physician's job is *then* not to think, but to oblige. Any physician of experience must have advised a patient against some unwise demand, and later received their gratitude. This commonplace experience renders the modern interpretation of the doctor's role wholly unacceptable. As we have shown, religious views are not to block curative medicine, as members of most religions would be eager to agree. But abortion and Euthanasia are not simple matters of curative medicine. They are complex ethical decisions where religious beliefs cannot but have relevance. Every informed person has a right and duty to express what he believes to be best for another's welfare, particularly if he is consulted in an area where the beliefs have relevance. Theistic faith is a highly contributary part of life. It cannot be arbitrarily amputated. The question of 'conscience clauses' will be discussed later. It cannot be stressed too much that what has just been said applies whether or not there is a 'conscience clause' available. A doctor's duty to advise his patient fairly obtains whether, or not, he is obliged to do what they request.

Christianity is largely concerned with motives. A Christian cannot ignore them in himself, or when they are plainly stated or can be inferred by others. He cannot *judge* these motives, but can and should recoil from sharing a motive which is 'self-centred' rather than 'God-centred'. He is also obliged to desist from sharing an act when the motive cannot be godly. For example, he could not assist someone to commit adultery.

Unfortunately the issues of motivation are not so simply solved. We have so far largely dealt with Christian *objections*. What is *a Christian's motivation* to be? This question has been reviewed by W. R. Matthews (who started with the motive of compassion), by many Catholic writers, who tend to argue from law via rules (e.g. the 'ordinary/extraordinary' distinction, 'the wedge', and 'double effect') and by Atheists who believe that there would be no problem had Christians not conditioned the world to faulty fears of death. Let us first look at these accounts.

(a) *Compassion as an argument for Euthanasia*

W. R. Matthews eloquently supported Euthanasia on the ground of Christian love and compassion (Matthews, 1969, p. 29). It is impossible to imagine any genuine Christianity which would not share that concern. But with all respect to such a scholarly Christian writer, we cannot see that this compassion can be so overriding as to justify so free an assumption of Divine mandate as Euthanasia, particularly when a satisfying alternative is possible, and when there are serious theological doubts about suicide. In this we are arguing that Matthew's approach had some parallels with the 'new morality' approach, where love is redefined so as to over-ride law, despite the fact that the apostle of love said, "sin is lawlessness" (1 John

3.4). Compassion is most important but cannot *necessarily* override law. (As an extreme example, consider some early Christian sects who killed their own children so that they might go to heaven and avoid a life of persecution. Few moralists have felt able to justify their action.)

Job's wife, no doubt concerned to end her husband's suffering, suggested a quick way out, "curse God and die". His exemplary refusal received the Divine approval. There is a Christian alternative to Euthanasia which Matthews barely mentions, compassionate intensive care (1 John 3.18). However, we do not aim to score in debate. Would that the compassion which Matthews so movingly described, and his evident sincerity, were enough to drive every Christian to renewed efforts to relieve suffering. We would also fully concede the Humanist case in the 'dignity versus vitalism' debate (J. Fletcher, 1969, pp. 61-70). It ought to have been the Christian case, and, if it were not so, Christians have failed to face the truth. It is no part of Christianity to preserve life *for its own sake.* It is, however, only fair to point out that it is a distorted caricature of Christian tradition which leads to preserving corporeal life 'at all costs'. Catholics have long rejected 'extraordinary methods' to achieve this, and other Christian traditions have held similar views. It is only when a truly Christian respect for life hardens into a rule of 'invariable sanctity of corporeal existence' that compassion fails and attitudes cease to be Christian at all.

Those who argue from compassion towards Euthanasia should remember that it must ultimately involve the decision of an outsider—the doctor—on the patient. Whether the patient leaves a document in advance of his illness, whether it is necessary to decide upon the sanity of his request, or whether his problem is one of diagnosis or prognosis, the decision and the compassion are finally in the doctor's mind. Thus the argument from compassion opens the door widely to *compulsory* Euthanasia, since it would surely be kindest to relieve those who cannot signify their wishes because they are disabled.

(b) *Morality by rule*

We have already mentioned the Catholic distinction between 'ordinary' and 'extraordinary' treatments. Another rule attempts to assess freedoms by the 'wedge' principle. This states that an act cannot be right for an individual if, were it widely practised, social evil would result. A third rule involves 'double effect'. Applied to suicide this would say, "when I relieve suffering, and in so doing happen to speed death, the action was licit if my motive was centred in relief, illicit if centred on speeding death"'

Such blanket rules are quite useful in abstract debate, but prove fragile in real life. We have argued against them elsewhere on this ground (Vere, 1969, 1967). For example, today's 'extraordinary measure' becomes ordinary (if it is successful) tomorrow, but not if it fails. The classification is thus arbitrary in practice, though very valid as a concept in abstract. The 'wedge' has been attacked as becoming a reason for doing nothing (Williams, 1957, pp. 280-281). Kamisar (1969, p. 115) ably defended it. Whilst conceding that "if a first step is moral, it is moral wherever a second step may take us", he goes on to show that whether or not a first step is moral depends in part upon what the second step is likely to be. In our view Kamisar is right, and Williams in error, since there is objective proof of the validity of that for which the 'wedge' model stands, if not for its naive application. (Daube, 1967, quoted German evidence that the promulgation of contraceptives diminished the incidence of abortion and vice versa, and that this effect can paradoxically *raise* the birth rate when contraception is made available. This is objective evidence of a case where decisions made for individuals have major outcomes for society.) It is a fact that attempts to secure esoteric freedoms for minorities can end by weakening broad and needful restraints upon the many, and may so evoke greater social evils. It is always necessary to consider the broad outcome of a narrow act, in so far as this is possible. The problem, and the weakness of the 'wedge' idea, is that we so seldom can foresee such outcomes. One thing is clear, that hopes centred in a good outcome from selfish humanity are bound to lead to false expectations.

'Double effect' is again weak in practice. Motives wear a little thin at times, as with the proverbial rabbit which ate its young to save them from the cat. For example, it is only too easy to expose a patient to a 'pound' of investigation to gain an 'ounce' of benefit. It is easy to choose a lethal starting dose of a narcotic to ensure that suffering will really be relieved.

Williams has mounted one of his most ingenious and misguiding attacks on current medical practice on the ground of double effect (1970, p. 665). Doctors, he implies, have used increasing doses of morphine to relieve terminal pain, and have either not noticed, or decided by double effect not to notice, that respiratory depression was speeding death. What will happen, he demanded, when new analgesics come which do not depress respiration? A doctor who used morphine then would be liable to a charge of murder.

First, he does not seem to understand *tolerance* (or tachyphylaxis) to a drug. This means that increasing doses are required to gain not only analgesia, but *also* respiratory depression. This is because tolerance develops to all the effects of opiates together, so that the dose required to depress ventilation rises with, and continuously exceeds, that needed for analgesia except in a very few people with respiratory insufficiency. This protects patients from serious respiratory failure provided the dose is slowly raised from a low starting level. What is more, when pain has been relieved by opiates, it is commonly noticed that patients begin to eat more and move about again. Though the normal effect of opiates is to depress appetite, pain can depress it more strongly, so that patients may improve physically once their pain has been relieved. So, contrary to common lay belief, opiates can *prolong* life rather than shortening it when skilfully used in suitable cases. (*Topics in Therapeutics*, 1978.) Hence Williams' damaging innuendoes that physicians are using Euthanasia now, though denying it by a dishonest trick, and could be scared out of the practice by the bogey of a murder charge!

No-one should be trapped by such devious arguments. Doctors no doubt once used morphine exclusively because nothing else was available, though used with ordinary competence it is still a valuable drug in the majority of cases. Recently, however, improved remedies, such as mixtures of phenothiazine drugs with opiates, abundantly demonstrate that suffering can be relieved without inevitably depressing respiration. No doubt, those who *wish* to induce Euthanasia may still use morphine in exaggerated doses for that purpose and so be at risk from the law. That is their concern; there is not the overwhelming reason to change the law for their sakes that Williams envisaged. He has used the fact that morphine can be used in more than one way, to delude us into thinking that a minority of the profession represents the practice of the whole (1970, p. 665).

In summary, enough has been said to show that rules, though useful in abstract debate, cannot furnish a helpful guide to practice. It is so easy to conceal, often unwittingly, a tangle of mixed motives beneath a rule. It is probably better to focus attention on motive. Once attention becomes focussed on a rule this comes to preempt all. When we try to simplify pleasing God by using rules, our weak hearts commonly end by pleasing the rule rather than God.

(c) *Christian conditioning*

This is a serious argument which undercuts all that has

been said so far, for we have accepted certain premises which this argument calls in question. It is contended that objection to suicide springs from a misconceived horror of death or of dying, which some do not hesitate to attribute to Christianity, or at least to Augustine's view of it. (Williams, 1970, p. 664; Barrington, 1969, p. 153ff.; Gillon, 1969, p. 176.) Gillon wrote "It is remarkable that whatever attitude was taken to the concept (of suicide) in general, for the purpose of voluntary Euthanasia it was always philosophically acceptable before the Christian era". It is also argued that the past 'theological era' produced a paradoxical fear of death—paradoxical because the theology should have led men to welcome death in anticipation of what lay beyond it (J. Fletcher, 1969, pp. 62-63, 68).

Were this view accepted, it would of course become absurd to analyse motives as we have done. Even an assumedly good motive leads to false ends if it is based on misinformation. However, we have been at pains to show that the Christian case did not arise, as Williams wrongly averred, when Augustine became frightened by the numbers of suicides among his flock, though their mistake no doubt crystallised his doctrine. It springs from Genesis 9 and from Job, and, as an obvious inference, from the extended teachings of Christ and of Paul about life and death. Augustine was too scriptural a theologian to have invented such ideas for himself *de novo*.

The fact is that Christianity conditions men to accept death, and to hope beyond it; but still to respect strongly God's control over life in areas where this has not been expressly delegated to men. This attitude was most clearly Paul's when he wrote—"For me to live is Christ, and to die is gain" (Philippians 1.19-26). Christianity prepares people to accept a truth which is broader than their own desires and sufferings.

Having dealt with such objections, rules and origins, it is possible now to ask what a true motive may be in regard to intolerable suffering. Proponents of Euthanasia advance compassion (e.g. Matthews, 1969), the aim to secure a dignified death (J. Fletcher, 1969, pp. 69-70; Gresham, 1969, p. 151), freedom and legal right (Downing, 1969, p. 22; Flew, 1969, pp. 30, 31) and progress (Williams, 1969, pp. 143, 144; Listowel, 1969, pp. 5-6). These motives have been reviewed with clarity and perspective by Waterson (1966).

Informed Compassion is integral with Christianity. The problem is how it should be shown. Compassion must be a leading motive, but it must be informed. It should not conflict with the revealed scriptural mandates. (Job's wife, no doubt, was as much concerned with compassion, freedom, dignity and progress, as were his comforters!) It should not merely transfer the burden of suffering and guilt from the patient to his relatives, friends or attendants. It should not damage the sufferer's communion with God. But it will strive at all practicable costs to ensure relief. This is where the Church may well have proved half-hearted. True, there are many pioneer Christian centres for the relief of suffering. (Are there any similar atheistic foundations?) Yet the awful burden of suffering is that the resources of knowledge and supply are so often not brought to those who need them. Far too many people in 'civilised' lands still die in loneliness and pain; not because resources do not exist, but because they are not mobilised for their benefit. This is urgent 'action-spot' for informed compassion today.

Freedom, progress and dignity are all desirable, given that their source and goal are defined. As words they are valueless. Pure, or essential freedom does not exist. The abolition of all restraints brings slavery to self. The imposition of wise restraints, based on man's 'design conditions', leads him into the freedom of a useful life, just as a train free from rails is useless, and water free from a glass cannot be drunk. Similarly, progress and dignity can only be defined by reference to concepts outside themselves, so that one man's progress is another's retrogression, one man's dignity is another's stultification. Such relative terms cannot be used to further any argument.

The only worthy motive is love, informed by God. Barrington (1969, pp. 160-161) remarked almost wistfully, in a very depressed and cynical essay, "Given superhuman love . . . there would be no problem. But the problem is there, and voluntary termination of life offers a possible solution that may be better than none at all." This is the thing in a nutshell. 'Given superhuman love'—that love exists, in Christ and through Him in His people. 'But the problem is there'—but so is the love! It is ineffective only in so far as Christians fail to give it to a needy world.

5. Euthanasia has both individual and social implications

Euthanasia, once practised, would certainly affect not merely individuals but also social attitudes to life and death. Its proponents are divided over this. Elliot Slater (1969, p. 58) argued "If we wish the human race to thrive, then we must accept the subordination of individual to racial values; we must acquiesce in the need for one generation to give place to the next". But, in the same book, Gillon quotes the Stoics to the effect that "Hegesias, the Cyrenaic, was so convincingly an advocate that King Ptolemy forbade him to lecture on suicide any more—too many among his audiences killed themselves after listening to him".

Presumably, there is a balance point somewhere in one's enthusiasm to give place to the succeeding generation. This gains a dimension in the question to what extent should such decisions be left to the individual, particularly in an over-populated world? Who may enforce his view on others? Many eloquent statements stress the voluntary nature of Euthanasia proposals; conscience clauses are put in every draft Bill of the type employed in the Abortion Act. But cheek by jowl with all this are statements to the effect that many should feel 'a sense of obligation' or be 'morally bound', to accept these very 'voluntary' proposals (Barrington, 1969, pp. 159-162). This seems rather inconsistent with the naive assertion that the proposals would be concerned "exclusively with cases where a patient is a burden to himself, and whether or not he is a burden to others plays no part whatsoever" (Barrington, 1969, p. 159). It seems that the new sense of moral obligation to accept Euthanasia will be voluntary because it will follow a social deconditioning from erroneous religious ideas.

The plain fact is that individuals, society and the conditioning process, are indissociable. Everybody is conditioned. There are no voluntary decisions in the absolute sense. The important thing, the battle for the mind, is to ensure that the bases of our conditioned decisions are true and valid. Pressures made by other people are not a valid base from which to decide.

Unvoluntary volition

Yale Kamisar (1969) exposed the bogus 'voluntariness' of Euthanasia in a most penetrating review. He asked "will not some feel an obligation to have themselves eliminated in order that funds allocated for their terminal care might be better used by their families?" The 'Voluntary' Euthanasia Bill (1969) comprised a clause (8) directing that certain treatments be given. Conscience clauses there are, but forceful pressure is exerted on those who use them, as in the attempts to persuade doctors to abort more freely (Scott, 1969).

The clash of ideologies

No one should blind himself to the fact that what we are seeing is not an issue of a voluntary kind at all. It is a battle between ideologies which condition men's minds and so partly govern their 'voluntary' decisions. The modern assertion is that atheistic 'freedom' should supplant religious conditioning. What nonsense; atheistic Humanism is itself a religion, with a basis of faith and a system of beliefs. The arbitrary decision (Gresham, 1969, p. 151) that "the effect of Euthanasia upon society, the family, the doctor . . . are secondary" is an arrogant assertion of one system of belief over another. Theists have become too readily brow beaten by those who arbitrarily rule their own ideas supreme, and claim that all religious argument is obfuscating. The truth cannot be gained by opposing one arrogance by another (see e.g. Worsthorne, 1970).

6. Euthanasia is concerned with laws

The *present British law* prohibits murder—or killing with an intent which is guilty, or causing any harm of a reckless or deliberate kind which leads to death. There is also manslaughter, the commission of an unlawful or dangerous act which kills someone, or the wanton or reckless neglect of a duty which leads to a death. No one has suggested changing this main intention of the law. Change is urged at a deeper level, that of the definition of the intention *behind* the law. Thus Williams (1970) argues that we no longer prohibit murder because it is 'wrong', but for reasons of 'secular morality, utilitarianism and empathy'. However, though Williams thus wants to weaken the very foundation of our law, he argues at other times from the full rigour of its existing sanctions to prove an imagined need to weaken its detailed prohibitions of Euthanasia as well. However, the law has not yet been changed in that way.* Exceptions have been made to cover cases of difficulty. These are either at the level of punishment of the guilty ('diminished responsibility' mitigations) or, more recently, an exception to the law itself (therapeutic abortion). It is Williams' case that a similar exception should be made for Euthanasia (Williams, 1970) on the grounds of the sufferer's rights, and the risk of a murder charge against the doctor who uses life-shortening narcotics to relieve pain. (It would, of course, be well nigh impossible to prove a guilty or negligent *intent* against the doctor, though the unpleasant charge could

* For the second edition of this booklet, a brief summary and discussion of the material relating to current proposals for changing the English criminal law has been included as Appendix I, page 55.

be brought with all its adverse publicity. Legislative change is urged to spare patients and doctors this adversity.)

The effect of weakening law

We should beware of such 'tubular vision'; it can be unwise to weaken a law which effectively protects many to assist a few. This is 'legislation on pretext'. It is precisely here that the Christian alternative appears. We will discuss this more fully in section 9. However, it has been shown that opiates can be combined with other drugs to relieve pain effectively without shortening life, provided that there is a programme of supportive nursing, free access to relatives and loving care (Saunders, 1959). Secondly, the only reason why these resources are not available to anyone is their faulty deployment, not that they do not exist. Given these therapeutic possibilities, it seems wrong to weaken by further exceptions a law which protects both fit people and the sick from other exploitations, and which conserves a healthy social respect for life.

This may seem doctrinaire, until the alternative is considered. Progressive weakening of law leads to increasing abuse. The 'slippery slope' argument is derided by opponents, but happens to be true in fact, as the abortion issue has demonstrated (see the House of Lords debate, 1969, columns 1159, 1191, 1192, 1177, 1205 and 1208). Small freedoms gained do lead to larger liberties in practice. Whether the gain is money, scientific knowledge or the satisfaction of a well meant but ill informed compassion, exceptions to law become heavily exploited. They may be justified if there is no practicable alternative. With Euthanasia there is a theistic alternative to the dogma of despair.

Need the law prohibit mercy-killing?

The existing law has been described as 'cruel and degrading' (Flew, 1969, p. 33). The whole argument, it is said, is polarised by the fact that a law *exists*. Thus it comes to centre round the question, "Why should the law be changed?" rather than the more fundamental query, "Why need there be a law against Euthanasia at all?" (Flew, 1969). This is very fair comment, and it becomes necessary next to see whether it is the law, or its customary application which is cruel and degrading. The answer appears to be neither, but rather the officially accepted legal interpretations of it. Apparently M. Hale and Mr. Justice Byles agreed that the law meant any life shortening, whether deliberate or inadvertent, to be guilty (Gillon, 1969, p. 185). Both interpreters apparently had deliberate life-shortenings in view; but why need anyone interpret the law so as to isolate pain relief from any other kind of medical treatment in this way? *Any* treatment may, at times, risk life. All surgery is in that category. Why is terminal care so different? It is because a difference has been forced by those who wish it so. There is nothing to suggest that any doctor could be held to have been 'reckless' if he withdrew a treatment which most, not even all, of his colleagues agreed to be ineffective.

There is no need to alter the present law, which has useful functions, or to introduce another.* It is not the law which brings cruelty and degradation; rather by preventing abuses it safeguards patients from practices which could become cruel and degrading. If misunderstanding of the law leads to the withholding of pain relief, or to needless efforts to prolong existence, it is medical education and practice which are at fault. Without the law murders could readily be disguised as euthanasias; guilty motives could readily become indistinguishable from true compassion (Kamisar, 1969, pp. 90, 92).

This leads directly to the question of rights and liberties in the face of laws.

* See Appendix I (page 55) on current proposals for changes in the English criminal law.

7. The liberal principle

The case against prohibition

We have argued *for* law to protect people from abuses, and *against* legislation which offers aid to minorities to the possible detriment of the larger public. How common would the abuses be? Is it right to breach the 'liberal principle' on such grounds? The 'liberal principle' (see Flew, 1969, p. 32) may be stated like this, 'the onus is on anyone who wants to prohibit an act to furnish a generally acceptable proof to support the prohibition'. As an illustration we might use the fact that many murders have been committed with axes. Should we therefore prohibit the sale of axes, because they provide an opportunity for abuse? Now, why should not the few who want to end a life of suffering, and those prepared to help them, be left to do as they wish?

This kind of argument has today been built up into belief in a human right—the 'right to die'. This implies the right to choose death as a free act. It is argued that if this choice were made in advance of illness, so as to be deliberate and collected, then it is worthy. It should be enacted when serious illness comes. This 'freedom' could, therefore, only be available to those who are capable of such decisions. It would be very much a right for the enlightened intellectual.

Such a freedom can only be contemplated if two things can be proved—that a 'right to die' really exists, and that its exercise will not be harmful to others. We strongly contest both premises. In a world where there is no agreed position concerning who has the right to live, it is absurd to introduce a 'right to die', as if that cliché had some firm or agreed substance. Please note that it is the concept of a 'right' which is under criticism here. It is not the concept that in some circumstances it is proper to allow natural death to take place that is under attack. Indeed, the very reverse is our argument; it is right that people should be allowed to live, and die, naturally. The moment of death should be in general neither accelerated nor delayed by meddlesome medicine (Twycross, 1978), though some very difficult cases have been described (cf. the Johns Hopkins Case, Rachels, 1975).

The risks of death acceleration to other persons, and society as a whole, will be discussed shortly.

First we must deal with the argument that the only barrier to this 'freedom' is religious. It is commonly said that Euthanasia is largely obstructed by Christian dogmas foisted on society by the minority who hold them. This is where the 'liberal principle' is invoked. Why not have Euthanasia even if it might be abused or perverted in a minority of cases?

After all, every act, even the good and merciful, is open to abuse, or may be mimicked with evil intent. For example, Christ was slain ostensibly for national security (in fact, it was really 'for envy' that He was delivered up). It is then asked: 'Should the pursuit of national security be proscribed because it was once so abused?' The expected answer is 'no', and the suggestion which follows is, by analogy, that we should accept Euthanasia even were it occasionally shown to have been abused. To this argument is added the innuendo that it is primarily those members of society who believe in a caring God who wish to retain the law as it now is; the suggestion being that they would do better to relax the law and rely more upon God's care! This is compounded with further suggestions concerning the undesirability of a group with such beliefs being allowed to use that law to curb the freedom of those who do not share the beliefs. There is a substantial case for Christians to answer here; but it is well to remember that, as part of God's caring,

He gave the law.

Let it be added to all this that the type of law which a modern 'civilised' society is prepared to accept differs from that which is familiar to Christians and Jews from the Old Testament. Modern laws are aimed to curb evils, defined with reference to man; Jewish law was aimed to promote righteousness, and that defined with reference to God. The Gentile laws stress the letters of a code. The godly Jew feared even unwitting breaches of the spirit of the law, indeed of the will of God. He lived in an earthly theocracy. The modern Gentile is not necessarily a member of Christ's heavenly kingdom. So Christians are held in an uneasy balance between the two laws, unable to *assert* theocratic principles over Gentiles, but bearing witness to their belief that it would be best, now and hereafter, for pagans to acquiesce in God's rule over their lives.

Let us then accept the 'liberal principle', but with certain riders. There is a difference between the imposition of theocracy (as Calvin's supporters may have attempted in Geneva) and urging men to comply with God's laws. It is a difference which is often inapparent to Christian and pagan alike. The concept is still difficult; a Christian cannot enforce his views, nor can he withdraw from society. Christ enforced His views upon no one, but showed how the truth would force itself into open minds, into society, until 'the salt' was effective. Christianity is and will be a real ingredient of society, and of social policies, whether their advocates like it or not. The crux is that, while we may certainly accept the liberal principle, we believe equally that we can show that the truth about man's nature and the possibilities of exploitation, demand that law should protect his life.

The case against acceptance of legalised Euthanasia

The reasons why the present law is needed do not depend on there being a theistic majority. They are these:

(a) *Adequate safeguards for a Euthanasia law cannot be achieved.** This is primarily because it would always be easy for guilty motives to simulate kindness. This demarcates Euthanasia from the example of the axe murder, discussed above. To press the illustration, no one wants to abolish axes to prevent abuse. When axes are so abused, the fact is obvious. Such a murder cannot simulate kindness, murder disguised as Euthanasia could readily simulate an act of mercy. And it is inconceivable that all kinds of pressures, real and imagined, would not come upon such people once it was possible to sign one's life away. That would not be *voluntary* euthanasia (Saunders, 1978).

(b) *Conservative attitudes to life would be weakened* in the community. Such an entailment was earlier denied; but now has become apparent in the case of abortion. The safety of the individual depends ultimately on a high respect for human life. This respect demands for its sustenance both the prohibition of Euthanasia and the urgency of pre-terminal care. It does not first involve two people alone, any more than any other pair of 'consenting adults' is alone. It influences relatives, dependents, professions, and society. No one lives to himself.

(c) *Humane pre-terminal care is a preferable and practical alternative* (Downing, 1969, p. 19). Care is available and the knowledge exists to provide it. Unhappily, in our society, false priorities ensure that at times and in places it is not available to those who need it, so generating a demand for Euthanasia. The priority is not to change the law, but to provide the adequate care in an humane and informed way. To provide Euthanasia would divert people to the belief that

* See Appendix I on current proposals for changes in the English criminal law: problems of providing adequate safeguards (page 55).

the problem was solved, so cementing the attitude of our care-less society into a harsh permanence.

None of these reasons is specifically theistic. All appeal to popular acceptance. But all consist well with theistic beliefs. The theist would reinforce them on these added grounds:

(a) Theism is a self-consistent system of belief which is based on facts and commends itself to reason. It is irrational to omit the Giver of life from consideration of His gift. If God be the source and sustenance of life we need stronger arguments than convenience or passing desires, before we can accept the deliberate ending of life on request.

(b) Liberty is always relative and does not exist in any pure sense. We have just shown that all men are linked to others by duty, responsibilities, and relationships. The theist goes further to say that man's liberty is continually narrowed by his own sin (Romans 6 and 7), which, though it is a theistic postulate, is also a practical observable fact. Thus a weakening of law, however seemingly appropriate for an oppressed minority, is in danger of exploitation by the disingenuous many.

(c) To take innocent life without a mandate is wrong, even with merciful intent.

8. Who would perform Euthanasia?

Medical involvement is inevitable

It is always assumed that it would be the medical or nursing professions which would be given the duty, and rightly so because more than the mere clinical atmosphere of the project is involved. Treatment is the doctor's and nurse's business. It is a challenge they may not shirk, even when new and elaborate therapies (such as renal dialysis) force them to modify their ways of life because of the demanding and time consuming nature of these forms of treatment (G. P. Fletcher, 1969, p. 84). Were Euthanasia desirable, only medical men could perform it properly, because only they would be equipped to consider the patient's person and life in a professional decision. They normally attend the sick, and they have the knowledge and ability to act in such situations.

A damaged professional relationship

But the deliberate ending of life is repugnant to most doctors. They have therefore the choice (cf. Ormrod, 1968) of accepting a task which they deplore or opting out to see a new cadre of technicians provided by society to execute its wishes. Tensions between profession and society would thus be strained to the detriment of all. The doctor's role is healing, not to be the suspected purveyor of death.

The answer to this objection is that Euthanasia would be brought only to those who wanted it (Gillon, 1969, p. 192). This is too facile. It requires little imagination to think how patient's attitudes would change once they came to think of doctors as wielding such powers and practices. Anyone, who doubts that a doctor's image may be changed by the work he has to do, should discuss the matter with a gynaecologist who has had to face the abortion problem.

A divided profession

It would be best, were society to insist on Euthanasia, for a second 'profession' to be established for the purpose. This, indeed, would be the inevitable result, for doctors would have to identify themselves as those who did, or did not, perform this duty quite early in the course of many clinical engagements.

9. What would be the alternative?

In a world where population pressure, with increasing numbers of elderly sufferers, is becoming the biggest of many related problems it is essential to provide a satisfactory alternative to Euthanasia. Otherwise it will be advocated, like war, as the only way out. This is not, however, to say that Euthanasia would solve the population problem effectively. We have already shown that it would suffice in this respect only for an intellectual élite, unless it were applied compulsorily or unscrupulously.

The elements of the alternative have already been stated. There are really three—

(i) a recognition that population control is a problem for the earlier, not the latter end of life, by control of conception.

(ii) a resolve to change therapeutics so that means are found to avoid the prolongation of a demented or grossly disabled corporeal existence. For example, almost no serious attempts have been made to develop prognostic indices—methods to predict the likely outcome after strokes, in Parkinsonism, and in diabetes. More progress has been made in coronary disease and cancer, but it is still slight.

(iii) national resources should be diverted towards 'intensive pre-terminal care'. Such methods have been developed and shown to be effective at several hospitals, including St. Christopher's Hospice.

It will be said that this is all uneconomic and wasteful, that people are not motivated to nurse the dying or disabled, and really want to produce wealth instead. This may be a true statement of our national life as it is; but it gives no reason why we should not aim to change it. Motivation follows a lead, so it is necessary first to decide what life is about—wealth or people? There is no natural reason why it should not be concerned with both. The incurable and the elderly exist as real people. Even were Euthanasia available most of them would not want it. Our duty is to improve their care.

10. Conclusion

Euthanasia, the easing of suffering by inducing death, has been proposed on grounds of freedom, progress and compassion. These grounds have been closely examined in their wider contexts and found to be wanting. The penalties incurred by adopting legal voluntary Euthanasia would much exceed the benefits. There is a positive alternative—which includes intensive pre-terminal care—which has barely been explored by society, but which has been shown to be effective. It would seem better to concentrate on that. Since our society is already in great difficulties from its past decisions about the control of life, it would seem most unwise in view of our existing weaknesses, to add to them some similar decisions about death. A radically new approach is required instead. This is only possible when the deeper significances of life and death are grasped.

Appendix I

RECENT PROPOSALS FOR CHANGES IN THE ENGLISH LAW RELATING TO EUTHANASIA AND KINDRED OFFENCES

Contributed by Nick Miller, M.A., M.Sc.*

At present in English criminal law any intentional act to terminate the life of another, even if the other indicates his consent, is defined as murder. The only defences to the charge of murder are certain rare cases of killing in the course of the prevention of crime, self-defence or defence of property and carrying out the sentence of the Court in execution. The penalty for murder is always life imprisonment under the Murder (Abolition of the Death Penalty) Act, 1965. In cases where death is caused in circumstances of diminished responsibility on the offender's part[1] the Court may find the offender guilty of manslaughter and any sentence, from a discharge to life imprisonment, may be imposed. Providing direct assistance to an individual seeking to terminate his own life constitutes the offence of assisting suicide (Suicide Act, 1961) which is punishable at present by a maximum of 14 years imprisonment. In all these cases, the Director of Public Prosecutions has to approve criminal proceedings and may occasionally waive them.

Both murder and assisting suicide (and their related penalties) have been the subject of detailed review and proposals for change. These are discussed below:

* This Appendix is based in part on work of the Shaftesbury Project's Crime, Law and Punishment Group, which is a multi-disciplinary study group of Christians working in the criminal justice system. The group submitted observations to the Criminal Law Revision Committee on its working paper on offences against the person in 1977.

Nick Miller, who convenes the Group, has a law degree and has spent several years in criminological research, including work on offences against the person.

1. Proposals Relating to Criminal Offences

Four different approaches need to be distinguished:

(a) The proposal to re-classify the offence of murder in certain cases as a new offence of 'mercy killing'.

(b) The suggested introduction of 'voluntary euthanasia' as an exception to the definition of murder.

(c) A number of proposals relating to the right to die and the incurable patient.

(d) The suggestion that the offence of assisting suicide be abolished.

(a) *Mercy Killing*

The Criminal Law Revision Committee (CLRC) in their review of offences against the person (August 1976)[2] put forward for public discussion a suggestion that a new offence of 'mercy killing' be created. This would apply to a person who "from compassion, unlawfully kills another person who is, or who is believed by him to be,

(i) permanently subject to great bodily pain or suffering, or

(ii) permanently helpless from bodily or mental incapacity, or

(iii) subject to rapid and incurable bodily or mental degeneration.

The defendant should have reasonable cause for his belief that the victim was suffering from one of the conditions mentioned in (i), (ii) or (iii) and consideration should be given to the inclusion within the definition of a requirement that the killing was with the consent or without the dissent of the deceased."

It must be emphasised that, unlike proposals for 'euthanasia', the CLRC *does not* suggest that the criminal law should be changed to exclude from criminal sanction altogether the taking of life of an incurable patient. It is concerned to establish in law the circumstances in which it should be recognised that the killing committed is distinguishable from murder. This proposal would reduce the penalty imposed on anyone found guilty of the specified offence (to a maximum of two years imprisonment: see section 2(b)).

A number of major problems of definition arise in relation to this suggestion which occur in considering all the proposals recently put forward which are discussed here. Among them are:

(i) 'From compassion'

While it would be necessary to ensure that the defendant's intention was not, for example, to speed up acquisition of an inheritance or to rid himself of an awkward relative, the requirement of the particular motive is most exceptional in criminal law and would be exceedingly difficult to prove or disprove.

(ii) 'Who is, or is believed by him to be . . .'

The question of how permanent and acute is the pain, suffering or incapacity may be very difficult to answer (see Chapter 2). Many people may know of patients who have been said by doctors to have a permanent, incurable or progressive illness where the prognosis has not been fulfilled, perhaps because of an incorrect diagnosis, or because of new medical knowledge or skill, or of courage and tenacity in the patient and those close to him.

(iii) 'Helpless' and 'incapacity'

These terms are particularly difficult to define. Many who can help themselves little can help others a great deal and there have been remarkable achievements in, for example, art and literature by seriously handicapped people.

(iv) 'Consent' and 'dissent'

This part of the CLRC proposal is the most contentious of all. Lack of dissent would be almost impossible to prove and consent would itself raise major difficulties of proof. Consent would provide some protection to the person who did not wish to die, provided he was sufficiently strong-willed to resist pressure, and would protect those who were too young or who, for some other reason, were unable to show their consent. For the apparently clear case of killing with the victim's clear understanding and assent to what was to be done, questions remain as to when this consent should be given (see reference, page 18). There are great dangers in giving consent in a time of acute pain because of the pressure of events, but equally, there are problems if consent is given in advance. How far in advance? Has there been a change of mind? How can a Court be sure that consent has been given if there is no document in the case? What effect may the giving of general consent in a document before the onset of an illness have on a patient, and on his relationship with those who knew about this consent such as his doctor or relatives?

These problems of definition, and a strongly critical response from a variety of sources, indicate that the CLRC's suggestion of a new offence may never be formally adopted in their final report on offences against the person, which is expected to be published in early 1979. However, elements of the new offence they put forward may be considered in relation to sentencing (see section 2(b) below).

(b) *Voluntary Euthanasia*

Three Bills have been introduced into the Parliament since 1936 seeking a new Act which would go further than the proposals outlined in (a) above. The most recent bill was introduced by Lord Raglan in 1969.[3] In Section 1 (1) a clause was proposed to make lawful the administration of 'euthanasia' (defined as painless inducement of death) by a physician to a 'qualified' patient who has made 'a declaration' which is 'in force'. A patient would be 'qualified' if in his or her case, being over the age of majority, two physicians (one of consultant status) have certified in writing that the patient appears to them to be suffering from an irremediable condition—i.e. a serious physical illness or impairment reasonably thought to be incurable, and expected to cause severe distress to the patient, or to render the patient incapable of rational existence. The 'declaration' referred to is a witnessed declaration made at least 30 days and up to three years before euthanasia is considered, though if re-executed preceding its original expiry date, it becomes valid during the life-time of the declarant. The Bill made it quite clear that there was no duty to participate in the euthanasia if the medical practitioners indicated that they had conscientious objections.

This proposal clearly goes beyond that of the CLRC in making the killing a *lawful* act, whilst stipulating that it could *only* occur in circumstances where an adult patient had indicated his consent and *only* at the hand of a medical practitioner. Some of the same problems of definition (e.g. as regards 'irremediable', 'serious', 'severe' and 'capacity for rational existence') identified in paragraph (a) above are again encountered here.

What is made more explicit in this Bill is the status of the patient's consent in the written 'declaration'. Without such a declaration no action could be taken: with a valid declaration being available, it appears that the medical practitioners could administer euthanasia even if the patient might in future be in a position to state that he did not wish such action to be taken.

This Bill did not succeed in the House of Lords[4] but it is interesting to note that the British Humanist Association and the Voluntary Euthanasia Society, which have advocated such proposals over a long period, used a national opinion poll in October 1976 to establish public reaction to a suggested change in the criminal law which was in many respects similar to the Bill's proposals. They asked whether legislation should be introduced which would allow adults to "receive medical help to a peaceful, immediate death, if suffering from incurable physical illness which is intolerable to them, provided such help has previously been requested in writing". 69% of a sample of 2,125 people who were asked whether they agreed with such a change said that they did agree, half of them strongly and half of them moderately. 17% disagreed (just over half of them strongly) and 14% said they did not know.

(c) *Incurable Patients and the 'Right to Die'*

In February 1976 Baroness Wootton introduced into the House of Lords an Incurable Patients Bill which goes less far than Lord Raglan's 1969 Bill.[5] It sought to establish in law the entitlement of an "incurable patient to whatever quantity of drugs may be required to give full relief from pain and physical distress" and for him to be "rendered unconscious if no other treatment is effective to give such relief". 'Incurable' was defined as being judged by two attendant physicians to be suffering without reasonable prospect of cure from a distressing physical illness or disability that the patient finds intolerable.

In Section 3 of the Bill, it was proposed that a written request by the patient not to have his life prolonged in the event of brain damage should be regarded in that event as a current refusal to be given such treatment. In other sections it was proposed that death by misadventure should be recorded as a verdict, if the patient died through an intentional overdose or other intentional act on his part, and that there should be no responsibility on medical practitioners to interfere in cases of attempted suicide.

In the debate in the House of Lords it was argued by several speakers that the Section 1 provision accorded with the best medical practice. As regards the proposals in Section 3 (which is in many ways similar to the proposal outlined in Lord Raglan's Bill) a number of the same problems of validity of the written request, and subsequent change of mind, and of the degree of incapacity required to make the pre-arranged refusal of treatment operative, would be encountered.

In a subsequent article,[6] Barbara Wootton has again argued the case for the introduction of legislation to permit legal declarations refusing medical treatment in specified future circumstances. She has suggested that the declarant could appoint an executor comparable to an executor of a will, who would (if satisfied after consultation with physicians that the conditions envisaged in the declaration were realised) take the necessary steps to ensure that the expressed wishes were carried out. Amendments to the Suicide Act to exonerate the executor and anyone assisting him would be required. She points out that what she terms 'Right to Die' Bills have been introduced in almost every American State legislature and in eight States such a Bill had become law by the end of 1977.

It should, however, be noted that it does not appear that any of this American legislation allows the medical practitioner to induce death: it is only concerned with the refusal of active medical treatment. In her article, Barbara Wootton takes the proposal beyond the mere refusal of medical assistance and suggests that the declarant should indicate whether "nature should be allowed to take her course without medical intervention" or whether he wishes to permit "humane termination of life".

As with both the proposals outlined above, the problems of deciding when such declarations are to have legal force remains. At what point does the declaration become operable? Are we sufficiently clear that incurable illness can be adequately defined? What sorts of treatment by medical and surgical means might be allowed or might be excluded? How might conflicts between the executor and the medical practitioners involved be resolved?

(d) *The Abolition of the Offence of Assisting Suicide in Certain Circumstances*

As stated above, the current position in English criminal law is that while the act of suicide itself is no longer a criminal offence,[7] assistance to an individual in terminating his own life has been retained as a criminal offence.

It has been argued that this offence should be abolished and this has been given added impetus by the recent case of Derek Humphrys, a journalist who in 1975 assisted the suicide of his wife, Jean.[8] Humphrys had pre-arranged that he would supply his wife tablets when she decided that she could no longer bear the effects of malignant cancer of the spine. Following the publication of his book and considerable media publicity, the Director of Public Prosecutions stated that he would not proceed with prosecution in this case.

It is difficult to establish how frequently such circumstances might occur, as in many cases they will remain undetected, in others they will be unreported and in others unproven. It is, however, clear that not all circumstances are necessarily analogous to the Humphrys case and there would be a need to retain the offence for less 'compassionate' involvement in suicide. The revision of the law to allow the 'decriminalisation' of the genuinely compassionate case would inevitably encounter some of the problems outlined in paragraph (a) above.

Summary

The proposals outlined so far can be set out in summary form ranging from the least radical to the most radical as follows:

(i) Ensuring the availability of drugs and the exoneration from medical care in some cases: Wootton 1976 Bill and subsequent proposal (1978).

(ii) Exclusion from criminal law of *bona fide* cases of assisting suicide in compassionate circumstances: Humphrys.

(iii) Exclusion from criminal sanction of *bona fide* cases of killing by physicians with consent of patient: Raglan Bill (1969), Voluntary Euthanasia Society (1976), Wootton (including proposals for an executor) (1978).

(iv) Creation of lesser offence of 'mercy killing' in any *bona fide* case where patient's consent is obtained: CLRC (1976).

(v) Creation of lesser offence of 'mercy killing' in any *bona fide* case without patient's consent: CLRC (1976).

2. The Penalties in English Criminal Law

The range of penalties currently imposed for murder, manslaughter or assisting suicide are set out at the beginning of this Appendix. It is clear at present that where anybody is convicted of murder, in whatever circumstances, the Court is bound to impose a sentence of life imprisonment. It has been suggested that to avoid this (in certain circumstances where the killing is done with the consent of the patient or otherwise in good faith) some convictions for 'manslaughter' in circumstances of diminished responsibility have been brought in. In other cases, the Director of Public Prosecutions may have exercised his discretion and waived prosecution.

Consequently, it has recently been argued that, failing a change in the substantive law to allow either euthanasia or a new offence of 'mercy killing', the mandatory penalty for murder should be abolished and a Court should be free to impose whatever sentence it deems fit. This, it is contended, would do away with any need to take account of tragic circumstances surrounding a particular killing where currently executive discretion may be exercised in releasing a convicted murderer on licence, after serving only a short term.[9] It is not clear how frequent such cases are. Only 50 murderers out of 590 released on licence between 1949 and 1976 have been released within a five year period, and only 12 of them within two years or less. How many of these may have been for offences akin to 'mercy killings' is not known.

Proposals which have been put forward recently for changing the powers of the courts in sentencing in relation to 'mercy killings' and kindred offences include the following:

(a) *Decriminalisation of euthanasia and certain cases of assisting suicide*

If legislation on the lines of Lord Raglan's 1969 Bill or of Barbara Wootton's 1978 proposals were passed, no criminal proceedings would be taken against medical practitioners intentionally terminating patient's lives. Equally, if certain compassionate cases of assisting suicide were excluded from criminal sanction, no sentence would be imposed on those who could show that their action came within the excluded category.

(b) *CLRC proposals concerning 'mercy killing' and tragic cases of murder*

In their 1969 working paper, the CLRC suggested that an offender found guilty of 'mercy killing' should be liable to a maximum of two years imprisonment.[10] Should this new offence of 'mercy killing' not be adopted, they suggest that in certain 'tragic cases' of murder (which fall within the scope of the suggested new offence) the trial judge should be given the power to impose a mental hospital order, a probation order or a conditional discharge. The judge would have to be satisfied that 'it would be contrary to the interests of justice for the accused to serve any sentence of imprisonment'.

(c) *Abolishing mandatory life sentences for all cases of murder*

The Advisory Council on the Penal System (ACPS) have recently reviewed maximum sentences in English criminal legislation. In their report[11] they propose that the current mandatory sentence of life imprisonment for murder should be altered to allow total discretion as to the sentence to be imposed (including the option of life imprisonment which would *only* be retained for the offence of murder). A similar recommendation was made by the Butler Committee on the Mentally Abnormal Offender.[12]

It is clear that such a departure from the mandatory life sentence would reduce the resort to the defence of diminished responsibility in cases of 'voluntary euthanasia'. It would also do away with the necessity for the apparent 'double-think' of the use of executive discretion in releasing a convicted murderer early in his life sentence under licence. Nevertheless, it is questionable whether the proposal for the change in the mandatory life sentence is appropriate. It can be argued that a life should continue to be 'taken' symbolically for the taking of the life of another person or, at the very least, that the offence of killing should be 'marked out' by a mandatory life sentence, however the effects of this sentence might be mitigated by executive discretion. The power to impose short terms of imprisonment or non-custodial penalties for killing in whatever circumstances may be felt to bring the law in to disrepute when compared with significantly longer sentences passed for other offences (notably property offences). The ACPS suggest that it is not clear that the public are in fact aware of a definite distinction in sentencing a murderer, particularly where life imprisonment is at present also used for other non-fatal offences. It can be argued, however, that the changes proposed might alter the public's perception of the seriousness of the deliberate taking of the life of another in whatever special circumstances. Views on both sides lack clear supporting evidence which might be provided by detailed research: this, by its very nature, might well only produce results which were equivocal.

(d) *Assisting suicide*

The CLRC in their 1976 report recommended the retention of a maximum sentence of 14 years imprisonment for assisting suicide. The ACPS however, suggested in their wider review of all maxima, that the statutory maximum should be reduced to six years imprisonment, though in certain cases (where by reason of the nature of the offence and character, conduct and antecedents of the offender, the Court was of the opinion that a custodial sentence of exceptional length was necessary for the protection of the public against serious harm) this maximum could be exceeded. The exceptional circumstances would probably be encountered very rarely in *bona fide* cases of compassionate assistance to a suicide.

3. Summary and Conclusions

It is clear that the issue of assisting a person with the ending of his life, either by helping him to kill himself or by the painless inducement of death, raises very significant problems in criminal law. These arise both as regards the definition of circumstances in which such conduct should be permitted and as regards the appropriate means whereby courts should deal with those involved in such cases. The discussion above will have shown how difficult it is to arrange the law and provisions for sentencing in a way which allows mercy to be shown in a truly tragic case, while providing clear protection for the most vulnerable, and maintaining the dignity of human life.

It is not clear that proposals for the making of declarations to ensure a 'right to die', or to allow euthanasia by a medical practitioner, can be adequately defined so as to avoid contentious cases. There is a considerable possibility of the law's falling into disrepute through its misuse and the lack of public ability to challenge 'borderline' decisions. On balance, therefore, we would conclude that from a legal standpoint, criminal offences as currently defined should stand, and that discretion as to medical intervention should be left to physicians as at present.

As regards sentencing, we have shown that there certainly are dilemmas in the operation of the system at present, though this probably occurs only in rare cases. The proposal to do away with a mandatory sentence of life imprisonment for murder seems likely to win considerable public support. As Christians, however, we would argue on balance that it is preferable that this sentence should be retained, albeit in a somewhat 'fictional' form through the use of executive discretion in 'tragic' cases. This, we feel, would be preferable to giving the courts total discretion as to sentence, and to the alternative outlined in Section 2 (b) above, which gives rise to significant problems in defining the exact boundaries of 'tragic' cases. We have no objection, however, to the ACPS suggestion that the maximum sentence for assisting suicide might in most cases be reduced, as in cases where the offender acted out of 'compassion' we are convinced that the Court would not avail itself of the maximum penalty, however long a period that might entail.

Footnotes and references

[1] That is, where the offender was 'suffering from such abnormality of mind (whether arising from a condition of arrested or retarded development of mind, or any inherent causes, or induced by disease or injury) as substantially impaired his mental responsibility for his acts or omissions' (Homicide Act, 1957, s. 2).

[2] Criminal Law Revision Committee, *Working Paper on Offences against the Person*, HMSO, 1976, paras. 79-87.

[3] The text of the Bill can be found in *The Unfinished Debate on Euthanasia*, H. Trowell, SCM Press, 1973, pp. 172-176.

[4] It was defeated by 61 votes to 40.

[5] The debate on the Bill's second reading can be found in House of Lords Debates, 12.2.76, cols. 196-214 and 226-302.

[6] *The Right to Die*, New Society, 26.10.78, pp. 202-203.

[7] Suicide Act, 1961, s. 1.

[8] See D. Humphrys, *Jean's Way*, Quartet Books, 1978.

[9] By the Home Secretary on the recommendation of the Parole Board after consultation with the Lord Chief Justice and trial judge (if available) under the Criminal Justice Act, 1967, s. 61 (1).

[10] Criminal Law Revision Committee (1976), op. cit.

[11] Advisory Council on the Penal System, *Sentences of Imprisonment: A Review of Maximum Penalties*, HMSO, 1978, Chapter 12.

[12] Report of the Butler Committee on Mentally Abnormal Offenders, HMSO, Cmnd. 6244, 1975.

Appendix II

AN ARGUMENT FROM THE THEORY OF KNOWLEDGE

There are more sophisticated arguments about prognostic error, of deeper theoretical relevance than those cited in section 2—that the possibility of error proves that no one ever *really knows* a disease to be incurable (Flew, 1969, p. 38), and the kindred theme that the severity of suffering must always be in doubt because it is immeasurable. Flew brilliantly showed that the first argument, that no one really knows anything, is metaphysical, and in every case not peculiar to Euthanasia at all. It would, if pressed, be an argument for never doing anything. "It is an inescapable feature of the human condition that no one is infallible about anything, and there is no sphere of life in which mistakes do not occur. Nevertheless, we cannot as agents avoid, even in matters of life and death and more than life and death, making decisions to act or to abstain. It is only necessary and it is only possible to insist on ordinary strict standards of warranted assertability."

Because he has shown that, in respect of prognostic certainty, Euthanasia decisions would not differ from any ordinary clinical decision, Flew argues ingeniously that we should go ahead and take them in the ordinary way. But Flew is here culpable, as one who from his standard of argument is certainly intelligent enough to know, of ignoring the very features of Euthanasia which we have discussed, which distinguish it from other classes of human activity in degree. The 'ordinarily strict standards' no longer apply here, though they may be helpful elsewhere.

Decisions affecting life and death are normally made with intent to cure, when there are no alternatives, and when evidence may later accrue to check the reliability of the decision. So they have a universally approved ethical substrate and means of verification. In short, doctors who treat patients with the aim of cure use two simple methods of self-correction. If they find their treatment is mistaken they change it, and if the patient dies from natural causes they may detect their mistakes at a *post mortem* examination. These methods cannot be applied to errors in Euthanasia, where the cause of death would be the patient's wish, and errors could be neither reversed nor corrected. These conditions do not hold good for Euthanasia. It is neither commonly approved nor is its aim restorative. Furthermore, its results cannot be validated in retrospect. We cannot therefore *really know* about Euthanasia as much as we can in ordinary therapeutic situations, whether the 'knowing' be ethical or scientific.

One of the commonest mistakes in argument by those who support or oppose Euthanasia is to compare things which are not strictly comparable. Flew's argument is a good example of this. The existence of a vague similarity of quality is not enough to warrant a similarity of practice. The argument that suffering need not be taken seriously because it cannot *really* be measured can also be successfully countered by Flew's ingenious first argument. It is, however, then complicated by the fact that feelings, being subjective, are not susceptible to normal scientific verification. They are always expressible only through the mind of *one* observer, the sufferer himself. We shall not pursue this here, save to point out that this uncertainty can and does at times contribute to diagnostic error. It is not a final argument *against* Euthanasia; there is plentiful evidence that some people die slowly in appalling distress. Nor is it an argument for Euthanasia; the request for death can always come only through one mind. It will therefore never be as verifiable as are objective criteria. Euthanasia is, in this sense, always requested on psychiatric rather than on physical grounds.

Appendix III

AN ARGUMENT FROM MODERN THEOLOGY

Recently, a new and significant argument has been adduced from Bonhoeffer's dictum that "Man has come of age" (MacKinnon, 1970). It is said that, as a matter of objective fact, man is now grown up in the sense that he has wrested so much knowledge from his environment, has modified his own living to such a degree, and has learned to decide about his problems rather than accepting all that comes to him, that his situation differs in kind from that of our early race. Bonhoeffer had, as a Christian, adduced this as a sign of man's growing maturity and conformity to Christ's image. A child must passively accept, a man should rationally choose. MacKinnon discussed the implications of this for human life and death, adding another premise, that it is right to pray for the dead in Christ that God's good work may be perfected in them. From these ideas he argued that all self-conscious decisions about life should be respected, but also, in the new situation in which man finds himself, decisions about death should be encouraged as part of the mature Christian's choice.

After discussion of conventional choices, MacKinnon puts the alternative, "Yet if others, more sensitive perhaps to the transformation in this present age in the ways in which men must see their relation to their environment, in full possession of their faculties, humbly before God, resolve in advance of the onset of such illness or of . . . senility, . . . that in face of such threats, they must be free to lay down the burden of their lives, their decision must also surely be respected. In both cases we must see that we are reckoning with a decision, with the self-conscious action of a man or woman who has 'come of age'." MacKinnon is concerned less with Euthanasia than with the theological principles that should govern our thinking about death. However, he saw a legislative outcome from these theories favourable to assisted suicide, and felt that Christians who had grown up spiritually in these ways would "find the impulse to mediate to their age the light which they claim to be particularly theirs".

MacKinnon's emphases upon death as a part of life, and as a part to be accepted, seem wholly admirable. Many impasses of suffering might be avoided were that idea learned and applied. It was also a new and helpful idea to apply Bonhoeffer's dictum to the problems of death to discover the outcome. However the attempt may be seriously misleading for the following reasons.

1. Attention becomes focussed on the mature Christian as one who decides, rather than blindly accepting what comes to him. As MacKinnon phrased it, we "take upon ourselves the burden of our human existence". The idea is excellent and the aim worthy, but the form misleads. Though a 'deciding maturity' is most evident in the Son of Man (Matthew 26: 43) and in His apostles (e.g. Philippians 1) in this very context of a choice of death, it is equally clear that their thinking did not start at that point. 'Man come of age' is not a primary Biblical doctrine, but is secondary. Antecedent to any decision, or ability to decide, came the revealed mandates which form the substrate of decision. It seems utterly clear (from the RSV of Matthew 26: 42) that Jesus was not merely deciding. He was deciding to do *God's revealed will for Him.* Thus, a truly Christian decision is independent only in the sense of being the resolve of an individual's will. It is, however, made in complete dependence upon the Divine purpose.

2. It was argued that we should respect all mature decisions, whether to accept suffering or to abandon life. But it follows from 1 that we should not 'respect' decisions just as such but only those whose maturity is proven in their demonstrable accord with God's will. We should, of course, respect the sincerity of those who decide even if they may prove to have been mistaken.

3. The antecedents of decision are at least as important as the ability to decide. Not all Christians would have chosen the antecedents used by MacKinnon, as he was ready to admit. Many would prefer to begin with revealed mandates of respect for life rather than dubious premises about prayers for the departed in Christ.

4. If the ability to frame mature decisions, important as it

is, becomes the pivot of our Christianity, several major defects are likely to afflict it. For example, the argument reduces to a form which might be caricatured to say "since many of our present problems arose from our past decisions about life, let us seek their solution by taking further similar decisions about death". Put otherwise, the danger is to use a situation which exists, because we have created it, to justify the selection of a theological position which fits it. This is then a concealed 'is' means *'ought'* argument. If Christianity means anything at all it must be that the world could have been otherwise. It is a radical critique of this 'world' which is part product of human decisions. The 'man is come of age' argument is a weak choice since it starts with the 'world' as it is, with human decisions as a good thing.

No one knows what the world might have been like given God-centred decisions; we know that it would have been very different. A similar problem is commonplace in therapy. Poor physicians add treatment upon treatment to correct the adverse effects of their earlier choices. Better men often stop everything and begin again. Similarly, it is our option either to say that we have learned to decide in life and so should now decide our deaths, or to decide radically to criticise the impact of medicine on life so that this becomes more godly, and then to see what is left of the problem of death. It seems likely that the residual problem would be much reduced, though it must freely be admitted that many intractable difficulties would remain. However, if we capitulate, allowing our situation to create itself, we have become victims of our own machine.

The contents of decisions also get insufficient attention when interest focusses primarily on decision itself. For example, it has been argued that decisions on death would be tantamount to those on life. This is not the case. If, in curative medicine, we decide to aid nature so that extra life is, in effect, given to someone who would otherwise have died, that new life is the life they would have lived had they not been spoiled by an evil disease. If, instead, they were to ask for induced death, that death would not have been their own death. In 'accepting' death in that way they would accept a death other than their 'own', and in fact reject the death (and life) which they were 'given'. This may seem a narrow point, but it has more validity. There are scriptural mandates for curative and palliative medicine, and for accepting death in a loving cause. There is no obvious mandate for death acceleration to avoid suffering or dementia or a sense of uselessness. There is therefore a real difference between 'accepting' life or death in these two situations.

It would therefore be best to preface application of Bonhoeffer's idea by consideration of the Biblical picture of man's maturity in Christ. Man *has* grown up, it is true, and this is a good and desirable thing. But it is in the sense that the prodigal grew up, taking what is his due, what had always been intended for him, but using it in a 'far country'. This resulted from a mature, respectable but self-centred decision. It is so noteworthy that his second decision was not to decide again as at first, but, "I will return to my Father". The solution was not a new infusion of wealth, but willing submission to the Father's decision for him. This was a more mature decision, an utterly independent recognition of true dependence. Maturity is willed submission. For Christ it meant "I do always those things which please the Father". For many mature and godly people down the centuries it has meant praying that they might die, if that were His will, rather than taking their lives.

There are in fact just two alternatives—to accept the Father's plan or to continue to let our chosen situation propagate itself. It seems likely that our better choice at present would be to ask how we may avert suffering more, by changing the policies and priorities of our medicine, rather than choosing an extended existence ended by an induced death.

So much for our therapeutic dilemma. There is also a theological dilemma for those who wish, as Christians, to "mediate to their age a light that they claim to be particularly theirs", at least in the legislative context. God-centred maturity is possible only to those who commit their lives to God. It is impossible to legislate for unbelievers on the basis of the deeper spiritual insights of a few Christians; even if their views agreed and were right they would still provide weak law for the many. Recently, several pieces of legislation have been effected on the pretext of the high ideals of the few. They have been miserably exploited by the many to worsen social problems rather than improve them. The point is that those who refuse to encounter God as Saviour must meet Him only in the moral law, which is applicable to all. Legislation cannot therefore be based upon the summits of individual piety but only upon mandates which apply to all. This need not prevent anyone from applying high standards to his own conduct within the law.

MacKinnon has done a real service in stimulating a new and enlightening debate. There is little that is new in this area from Christian writers. But we believe that his practical suggestions are the reverse of what should be done, self-consistent though they are within the very limited and somewhat dubious terms of reference.

References

Ailwyn, Lord (1969). In the House of Lords Debate, q.v.

Alexander (1949). Medical Science under Dictatorship. N.Eng. J.Med. 241, 131-132.

Barrington, M. R. (1969). Apologia for suicide, in Euthanasia, and the Right to Death. Ed. A. B. Downing; Peter Owen, London, 1969.

Brit.Med.J. (1978). Diagnosis of Brain Death. (Statement by the Secretary of the Conference of Medical Royal Colleges in the United Kingdom, 11 October 1976) British Medical Journal (1976) **2**, 1187-1188.

Calvin, J. (1536). Institutes of the Christian Religion. Republished in 1953 by Henry Beveridge, James Clark, London.

Chudleigh, Lord (1969). In the House of Lords Debate, q.v.

Clark-Kennedy, A. E. (1969). Moral Problems and Medical Practice. Nursing Times, Sept. 18th, 1969, pp. 149-152.

Daube, D. (1967). The Sanctity of Life. Proceedings of the Royal Society of Medicine, 60, 1235-1239.

Downing, A. B. (1969). Euthanasia: The Human Context in Euthanasia and the Right to Death. Ed. A. B. Downing; Peter Owen, London.

Dyck, A. J. (1977). On human care. An introduction to ethics. Abingdon, Nashville. ISBN 0 687 28845 2.

Explanatory Memorandum to the Voluntary Euthanasia Bill (1969) *ibid.*

Fletcher, J. (1969). The Patient's Right to Die, *ibid.*

Fletcher, G. P. (1969). Prolonging life; Some Legal Considerations, *ibid.*

Flew, A. (1969). The Principle of Euthanasia, *ibid.*

Giertz, G. B. (1966). Ethical Problems in Medical Procedures in Sweden. In Ethics in Medical Progress. CIBA Foundation Symposium. J and A. Churchill, London.

Gillon, R. (1969). Suicide and Voluntary Euthanasia. Historical Perspective, *ibid.*

Gresham, G. A. (1969). 'A Time to be Born and a Time to Die,' in Euthanasia and the Right to Death. Ed. A. B. Downing; Peter Owen, London.

House of Lords Debate on the Voluntary Euthanasia Bill (1969). Hansard 300, No. 50, Columns 1143ff.

Kamisar, Y. (1969). Euthanasia Legislation: Some Non-Religious Objections. In A. B. Downing, *ibid.*

Listowel, Lord (1969). Foreword, in A. B. Downing, *ibid.*
Longford, Lord (1969). In the House of Lords Debate, q.v.
McCormick, R. A. (1974). To Save or Let Die. J.Amer.Med. Assoc., 229, 172-176.
MacKinnon, D. M. (1970). Death as Part of Life. Crucible, July 1970, pp. 99-103.
Matthews, W. R. (1969). Voluntary Euthanasia: The Ethical Aspect, *ibid.*
Millard, C. K. (1931). The Case for Euthanasia. Fortnightly Review, 136: 701.
Miller, N. (1978). Murder or mercy, Third Way, pp. 7-9.
Ormrod, Sir Roger (1968). Medical Ethics. Brit.Med.J. April 6th, pp. 7-10.
Platt, Lord (1970). Euthanasia. Proc.Roy.Soc.Med. 63, 659-661.
Rachels, J. (1975). Active and passive Euthanasia. New England J.Medicine, 292, 78-80.
Russell, R. O. (1977). Freedom to Die: Moral and legal aspects of Euthanasia. Human Sciences Press, London.
Saunders, C. S. (1959). The Care of the Dying. London. Macmillan.
Saunders, C. S. (1978). World Medicine (Sept. 20th), p. 46.
Scott, J. S. (1969). Interpreting the Abortion Act. Lancet, Sept. 27th, p. 694.
Silverman, D. and others (1969). Cerebral Death and the Electro-encephalogram. J.Amer.Med.Assoc. 209, 1505-1510.
Slater, E. (1969). Death, the Biological Aspect. In Euthanasia and The Right to Death, Ed. A. B. Downing; Peter Owen, London.
Soper, Lord (1969). In the House of Lords' Debate, q.v.
Topics in Therapeutics (4) (1978). Chapters on the use of drugs and other treatments in pre-terminal care. Ed. D. W. Vere. Pitman Medical, Tunbridge Wells.
Twycross, R. (1978). The dying patient, CMF, London.
Vere, D. W. (1963). Errors of Complex Prescribing. Lancet.
Vere, D. W. (1967). Why the Preservation of Life? In Ethical Responsibility in Medicine. Ed. Edmunds, V. and Scorer, C. G. E. & S. Livingstone, Edinburgh.
Vere, D. W. (1969). Problems of Abortion and Sterilisation in Birth Control and the Christian; Tyndale House.
Voluntary Euthanasia Bill (1969), quoted as an Appendix by A. B. Downing, *ibid.*
Waterson, A. P. (1966). Medical Ethics: A Christian View. Ed. Edmunds, V. and Scorer, C. G., Tyndale Press (pp. 48-53).
Williams, D. (1978). A medicine called hope. Third Way, Jan. 26th, pp. 3-6.

Williams, G. (1957 NY). The Sanctity of Life and the Criminal Law. Faber and Faber, London, 1958.
Williams, G. (1970). Euthanasia. Proc.Roy.Soc.Med. 63, pp. 659-670.
Wolbarst, A. L. (1939). The Doctor looks at Euthanasia. Medical Record, May 17th, 149, 354.
Worsthorne, P. (1970). Labour a Slave to Minorities. Sunday Telegraph, May 31st.